Jokes For Elderly The Punch Line is in the Wrinkles

A Side-Splitting Book of Jokes for Seniors

Charlie Jacobs

Table of Contents

Introduction

Laughing is an essential part of life that brings people together, breaks down barriers, and promotes overall well-being. As we grow older, finding reasons to laugh becomes even more important, especially when life's challenges can seem overwhelming. That's why we have compiled this collection of jokes specifically tailored for the elderly.

Whether you're sharing a laugh with friends and family or just looking for a good chuckle to brighten your day, these jokes will provide you with plenty of opportunities to smile, giggle, and maybe even belly laugh. From classic one-liners to clever wordplay, these jokes are guaranteed to bring a smile to your face and a warmth to your heart.

We believe that laughter is the best medicine, and we hope that this book will provide you with a dose of joy and happiness whenever you need it. So sit back, relax, and get ready to laugh your way through this collection of jokes for the elderly.

Senior Moment

Two elderly gentlemen were sitting on a park bench when one turned to the other and said, "You know, I'm getting so forgetful in my old age, I can't even remember my own phone number!"

The other man replied, "That's nothing, I can't even remember my own name!"

They both laughed and then the first man asked, "What do you think we should do?"

The second man thought for a moment and then said, "Let's swap phone numbers, that way we'll at least have a chance of getting in touch with each other."

The Birthday Present

An elderly man was celebrating his 90th birthday and his friends and family had gathered to throw him a party. As he was opening his presents, he came across a small package from his wife.

Excitedly, he opened it up and inside was a small box with a pill in it. Confused, he turned to his wife and asked, "What's this for?"

His wife smiled and replied, "It's a Viagra pill, dear. You know what it's for."

The man laughed and exclaimed, "Wow, I'm 90 years old and you still want me to go at it like a young man!"

The partygoers all laughed and the man's wife replied, "Well, I just wanted to make sure you have a happy birthday!"

The Sneeze

An elderly woman walked into her doctor's office and said, "Doctor, I have a problem with uncontrollable gas. Luckily, the gas is always silent and odorless, but I can't seem to stop it from happening."

The doctor listened to her concerns and prescribed some medication to help alleviate the problem.

A few days later, the woman returned to the doctor's office and said, "Doctor, your medicine has helped with the gas problem, but now I have a new problem. Every time I sneeze, I pass gas loudly and uncontrollably!"

The doctor thought for a moment and replied, "Well, I think we'll have to adjust your medication. Let's see if we can get you fart-antihistamines."

The Elderly Couple

An elderly couple was sitting on their porch, enjoying the sunset and reminiscing about the past. The wife turned to her husband and said, "Do you remember the first time we had sex, dear?"

The husband thought for a moment and replied, "Yes, I do. It was right here on this porch, in fact."

The wife smiled and asked, "And do you remember how we did it?"

The husband chuckled and said, "Yes, I do. We did it standing up."

The wife looked surprised and asked, "Really? That must have been uncomfortable."

The husband smiled and said, "Not really. I was just leaning against the fence."

The Talking Parrot

An elderly woman decided to buy a talking parrot to keep her company. She brought the parrot home and spent hours trying to teach him how to talk. Finally, after many attempts, the parrot spoke up and said, "Hello, pretty lady!"

The woman was thrilled and said, "Thank you, parrot! Can you say anything else?"

The parrot thought for a moment and then replied, "Yes, I can. I noticed that you have a beautiful house, and I have to say, it's quite big for just the two of us."

The woman was taken aback and asked, "What do you mean, just the two of us?"

The parrot replied, "Well, I was just wondering if you're expecting any company. Maybe someone to clean up all this bird poop?"

The Forgetful Husband

An elderly couple was sitting down to dinner when the husband suddenly exclaimed, "Oh no, I think I left the stove on!"

The wife rolled her eyes and said, "Oh, you always forget something. Let me go check."

She walked to the kitchen and immediately smelled something burning. She turned off the stove and called out to her husband, "You left the stove on, but don't worry, I turned it off."

The husband replied, "Oh, good. While you're up, can you make me a sandwich?"

The wife sighed and said, "What do you say?"

The husband thought for a moment and then replied, "Thank you for turning off the stove."

The Smart Dog

An elderly man had a pet dog that he loved dearly. One day, the man went to the pet store and asked the owner if he had any smart dogs. The owner said, "As a matter of fact, I do. This dog right here can speak two languages and solve complex math problems."

The man was impressed and decided to buy the dog. He brought it home and immediately put it to the test. He asked the dog, "What's two plus two?"

The dog replied, "Four."

The man was amazed and said, "Wow, you really are a smart dog!"

The dog replied, "I'm not a smart dog. I'm just really good at math."

The Speeding Ticket

An elderly woman was driving down the highway when she was pulled over by a police officer for speeding. The officer approached her car and asked for her license and registration. After reviewing her documents, the officer said, "Ma'am, do you know how fast you were going?"

The woman replied, "I'm sorry officer, I don't. I didn't see any signs."

The officer said, "Well, you were going 80 miles per hour in a 55 mile per hour zone. That's a hefty fine."

The woman sighed and said, "Oh no, I can't afford that. Is there anything I can do to reduce the fine?"

The officer thought for a moment and said, "Well, there is one thing. Do you have anything to say for yourself?"

The woman replied, "Yes, actually. Last week my husband ran off with a police officer, and I thought you were trying to bring him back."

The officer chuckled and said, "Alright, I'll let you off with a warning this time. But please, slow down."

The woman smiled and said, "Thank you, officer. I'll try."

The Golf Game

An elderly man was out playing golf with his wife one day. On the first tee, the man hit a perfect shot straight down the fairway. As they walked towards the ball, the man turned to his wife and said, "You know, honey, when I was your age, I could hit the ball a hundred and fifty yards."

His wife replied, "Really? When I was your age, I could get the ball in the hole in one shot."

The man chuckled and said, "Well, I guess things change as we get older."

They continued playing and on the second tee, the man hit a poor shot that went off course. As they walked towards the ball, the man turned to his wife and said, "You know, honey, when I was your age, I could hit the ball straight as an arrow."

His wife replied, "Really? When I was your age, I could see where the ball was going even without my glasses."

The man laughed and said, "Well, I guess things change as we get older."

As they approached the third tee, the man hit the ball straight into a sand trap. As they walked towards the ball, the man turned to his wife and said, "You know, honey, when I was your age, I could get out of this trap in one shot."

His wife replied, "Really? When I was your age, that sand trap wasn't even here!"

The Wise Old Monk

A wise old monk lived high in the mountains and was known to have the answers to life's most challenging questions. One day, a young man decided to climb the mountain to seek the monk's wisdom.

After a long and difficult journey, the young man finally reached the top and met the monk. "Master," he asked, "What is the meaning of life?"

The wise old monk thought for a moment, then replied, "Life is like a bowl of soup."

The young man was confused and asked, "What do you mean?"

The monk continued, "You see, life is made up of many different ingredients, just like a bowl of soup. Some ingredients are sweet, some are sour, some are savory, and some are bitter. But when you mix them all together, you get a delicious soup that nourishes your body and soul."

The young man nodded, impressed with the monk's wisdom. "But what about the spoon?" he asked.

The monk smiled and replied, "The spoon is your journey through life. It's up to you to use it to taste and savor all the different ingredients life has to offer. And when the soup is gone, the spoon remains. So, make sure you use it wisely."

The Unhappy Parrot

An elderly man walked into a pet store looking for a companion. He spotted a beautiful, colorful parrot and asked the store owner about it.

The store owner warned him, "That parrot is beautiful, but he has a problem. He used to live in a bar, and he's picked up some bad language. So, if you have children or grandchildren around, it might not be the best fit."

The man was undeterred and decided to take the parrot home with him.

A few days later, the man returned to the store, looking quite unhappy. The store owner asked him what was wrong.

"I'm sorry to say that the parrot isn't working out. He keeps swearing and saying inappropriate things all the time," the man replied.

The store owner was surprised and asked, "Did you try talking to him or teaching him some new words?"

The man replied, "Well, I did try. I sat down with him and tried to teach him some new words. But every time I said something, he just looked at me like I was crazy."

The Wise Barber

An elderly man walked into a barbershop and asked the barber, "How much for a haircut?"

The barber replied, "Ten dollars."

The man asked, "And how much for a shave?"

The barber replied, "Five dollars."

The man nodded and said, "Okay, then. I'll be back tomorrow."

The next day, the man returned to the barbershop and the barber asked, "Are you here for a haircut or a shave?"

The man replied, "Both, please."

The barber nodded and began to work. After a while, the man fell asleep in the chair.

The barber finished and woke the man up, saying, "Sir, you fell asleep. Are you okay?"

The man replied, "Yes, I'm fine. I just wanted to

rest my eyes a bit."

The barber smiled and said, "Well, you're a wise man. You saved five dollars by sleeping during your shave."

The Lost Parrot

An elderly woman was heartbroken when her pet parrot flew out of the window and got lost. She searched everywhere for him, but he was nowhere to be found.

One day, she saw a young man with a parrot in his hand and she thought it might be her lost bird. She ran up to him and asked, "Excuse me, sir, is that my parrot?"

The man replied, "I'm sorry, ma'am, but this is my parrot. I bought him at the pet store."

The woman didn't believe him and said, "No, no, I'm sure that's my bird. He has a very distinctive feature. Whenever he speaks, he starts with 'Praise the Lord'."

The man looked at the parrot and said, "Let me try something." He then turned to the bird and said, "What's two plus two?"

The parrot replied, "Four."

The man then said, "And what's the capital of

France?"

The parrot replied, "Paris."

Finally, the man said, "And who is the Son of God?"

The parrot replied, "Praise the Lord!"

The Forgetful Senior

An elderly man walks into a doctor's office and says, "Doctor, I can't remember anything! I forget names, faces, even my own address."

The doctor replies, "How long has this been going on?"

The man says, "How long has what been going on?"

The Clever Waiter

A man walks into a restaurant and sits down at a table. He asks the waiter for a cup of coffee without cream.

The waiter replies, "I'm sorry, sir, but we're out of cream. Would you like it without milk instead?"

The Talking Dog

A man sees a sign outside a house that says "Talking Dog for Sale." Intrigued, he rings the doorbell and the owner brings out a dog.

"Can your dog really talk?" the man asks.

"Sure can," says the owner. "Go ahead, ask him a question."

The man asks the dog, "What's on top of a house?"

"Roof!" replies the dog.

The man asks another question, "How does sandpaper feel?"

"Rough!" replies the dog.

The man is amazed and decides to buy the dog. He takes him home and shows him off to his family and friends.

But after a while, the man starts to get suspicious. "Maybe the dog isn't really talking," he thinks. "Maybe the owner taught him to respond to certain questions."

So he decides to test the dog. He takes him to a pond and asks, "What's on top of a tree?"

The dog looks up and says, "Woof!"

The Hilarious Traffic Jam

A man is stuck in traffic and sees a priest walking on the side of the road. The man rolls down his window and calls out to the priest, "Father, can you do something about this traffic? I'm going to be late for my meeting!"

The priest nods and walks up to the front of the line of cars. He raises his arms and starts to pray. Suddenly, the traffic starts to move, and the cars ahead of the man begin to clear out of the way.

Amazed, the man rolls down his window again and yells out to the priest, "Father, you did it! How did you clear the traffic so quickly?"

The priest smiles and replies, "I haven't moved a single car. I just blessed the road ahead, and everyone else decided to make way!"

The Smart Lawyer

A lawyer was cross-examining a witness on the stand in a courtroom. He asked the witness, "Isn't it true that you were at the scene of the crime when it happened?"

The witness replied, "No, I wasn't there."

The lawyer smirked and said, "Well then, if you weren't there, how do you know what happened?"

The witness looked at the lawyer and said, "The same way you know that I wasn't there."

The Fisherman's Wish

A fisherman was out at sea when he caught a magical fish. The fish begged the fisherman to spare its life, promising to grant him three wishes in return.

Excited at the prospect of making his dreams come true, the fisherman quickly made his first wish. "I wish to be rich beyond my wildest dreams," he said.

The fish granted his wish, and the fisherman found himself surrounded by piles of gold and riches beyond his imagination.

For his second wish, the fisherman asked to be reunited with his long-lost love. The fish granted his wish, and the fisherman was soon holding his beloved in his arms.

Overjoyed at his good fortune, the fisherman struggled to think of what to wish for with his final wish. Finally, he turned to the fish and said, "I wish for a bottomless beer mug that never runs out."

The fish granted his wish, and the fisherman happily filled his mug with beer and drank until he was completely drunk.

As he stumbled home, he realized the mistake he had made. He could have wished for anything, and yet he had wasted his final wish on something so trivial.

The Talking Parrot

A man walked into a pet store and saw a parrot for sale. The parrot had a sign that read, "This parrot can speak English, Spanish, and French."

Excited, the man asked the pet store owner to demonstrate the parrot's abilities. The pet store owner said, "Sure, but be careful what you say. This parrot has a bit of a foul mouth."

The man agreed and the pet store owner started speaking to the parrot in English. The parrot replied in perfect English, shocking the man.

Next, the pet store owner spoke to the parrot in Spanish, and once again, the parrot responded flawlessly.

Finally, the pet store owner spoke to the parrot in French. The parrot looked at the man and said, "Excusez-moi, monsieur, mais je ne parle pas le français." (Excuse me, sir, but I don't speak French.)

The Cowboy's Horse

A cowboy rode into town on his trusty horse and went into the saloon for a drink. After a few too many, he stumbled outside and found that his horse had wandered off.

Determined to find his horse, the cowboy searched all night long. Just as the sun began to rise, he spotted his horse in the distance, grazing peacefully.

Relieved and exhausted, the cowboy staggered up to his horse and slurred, "I don't blame you for wandering off. I would have done the same if I had a horse like me."

The Talking Dog

A man walks into a bar with his dog and says to the bartender, "I bet you $100 that my dog can talk."

The bartender, thinking the man is crazy, decides to take the bet. The man turns to his dog and asks, "What's on top of a house?" The dog replies, "Roof!"

The bartender is unimpressed and tells the man to leave. As they walk out, the dog turns to his owner and says, "Do you think I should have said 'ceiling' instead?"

The Golf Game

Two friends were playing golf when one of them hit a terrible shot and it landed in a pond. Frustrated, he turned to his friend and said, "I don't think I can play anymore. This game is too hard."

His friend replied, "Don't worry, I have an idea. Just pretend that the pond is the ocean, and you're a pro surfer."

Feeling a little silly, the man agreed and took his shot. To his surprise, the ball skipped across the water and landed on the green.

Ecstatic, he turned to his friend and said, "Wow, that was amazing! What's your secret?"

His friend replied, "Oh, it's easy. Just remember, the ball doesn't know it's supposed to sink."

The Doctor and the Ghost

A doctor walks into a patient's room and says, "I have some good news and some bad news. The bad news is that you have a rare and incurable disease. The good news is that we named it after you."

Suddenly, the patient's ghost appears and says to the doctor, "I don't understand. How could you give him my name?"

The Fortune Teller

A woman goes to see a fortune teller and asks, "What do you see in my future?"

The fortune teller responds, "I see that you'll be married five times."

The woman is shocked and asks, "Will I really be married five times?"

The fortune teller shrugs and says, "I'm not sure. That's just what I see in my crystal ball. Maybe you'll marry the same man five times."

The Smart Parrot

A woman bought a parrot that she was told was very smart. One day, while she was out, a burglar broke into her house. The parrot, seeing the burglar, said, "Hey, you! Get out of here!"

The burglar was surprised and asked the parrot, "Did you just talk?"

The parrot replied, "Yes, I did. Now get out of here before I call the police!"

The burglar laughed and said, "What kind of a parrot are you? You're supposed to be smart."

The parrot replied, "I may be a parrot, but at least I'm not a burglar."

The Talking Dog

A man walks into a bar with his dog and says to the bartender, "I bet you $100 that my dog can talk."

The bartender looks at the man skeptically and says, "Okay, you're on."

The man turns to his dog and says, "What's on top of a house?"

The dog barks, "Roof, roof!"

The man then asks, "What's the opposite of smooth?"

The dog barks, "Ruff, ruff!"

The bartender, amazed, hands over the $100 to the man. As they leave the bar, the dog turns to the man and says, "You know, I should have said 'ceiling' instead of 'roof'."

The Three Wishes

A man finds a magic lamp and rubs it, and a genie appears. The genie says, "I will grant you three wishes, but be careful what you wish for."

The man thinks for a moment and says, "Okay, for my first wish, I want a bottomless mug of beer."

Poof! A bottomless mug of beer appears in front of him, and he starts drinking.

For his second wish, he says, "I want to be rich beyond my wildest dreams."

Poof! The man is suddenly surrounded by piles of gold and jewels.

For his final wish, the man says, "I want to be irresistible to women."

Poof! The genie turns him into a box of chocolates.

The Magic Mirror

A man walks into a bar and sees a sign that says "Free Drinks if You Can Make My Horse Laugh". He decides to give it a try and asks the bartender to take him to the horse.

The bartender takes the man to the horse, which appears to be in a bad mood. The man whispers something in the horse's ear, and it suddenly starts laughing hysterically.

The bartender, amazed, asks the man, "What did you say to the horse?"

The man replies, "I told him my salary."

The bartender, confused, asks, "How did that make him laugh?"

The man answers, "I also told him yours."

The Smart Parrot

A man goes to a pet store to buy a parrot. The salesman shows him a beautiful parrot and says, "This parrot is very smart. He can answer any question you ask him."

The man is impressed and decides to buy the parrot. When he gets home, he decides to test the parrot's intelligence. He asks the parrot, "What's two plus two?"

The parrot responds, "Four."

Impressed, the man asks, "What's the capital of France?"

The parrot responds, "Paris."

The man is amazed and decides to ask a more difficult question. He asks, "What's the meaning of life?"

The parrot responds, "42."

The man is confused and asks, "How do you know that?"

The parrot responds, "I read it in 'The Hitchhiker's Guide to the Galaxy'."

The Doctor's Diagnosis

A man goes to the doctor and complains of feeling tired all the time. The doctor runs a battery of tests and examines him thoroughly.

After all the tests are done, the doctor says to the man, "I'm sorry to tell you this, but you have a rare disease that is incurable and will cause you to feel tired all the time. You only have six months to live."

The man is devastated and asks the doctor, "Is there anything I can do to make the most of my last six months?"

The doctor responds, "Well, you could move to the countryside, go fishing, read books, and spend time with your family."

The man thinks about it for a moment and then asks the doctor, "Would that make me live longer?"

The doctor responds, "No, but it will make the six months feel like an eternity."

The Barbershop Quartet

A man walks into a barbershop and asks the barber, "Can you give me a haircut like the Three Stooges?"

The barber responds, "I'm sorry, I don't know who they are."

The man is surprised and says, "How can you not know who the Three Stooges are? They're famous!"

The barber responds, "Well, I'm not from around here. Where are they from?"

The man responds, "They're from America."

The barber says, "Oh, I see. You mean Larry, Moe, and Curly. Why didn't you say so?"

The man says, "Yes, that's who I mean. Can you give me a haircut like them?"

The barber says, "Sure, but it's going to cost you an arm and a leg."

The man is taken aback and says, "Why so much?"

The barber responds, "Well, you asked for a Three Stooges haircut, so I have to charge you for four haircuts."

The Lost Tourist

A tourist in Paris is lost and desperately trying to find his way back to his hotel. He stops a local and asks, "Excuse me, do you speak English?"

The local responds, "Yes, I do. How can I help you?"

The tourist says, "I'm trying to find my way back to my hotel. It's called the Hotel de la Paix. Do you know where it is?"

The local responds, "I'm sorry, I don't know where that hotel is."

The tourist is frustrated and says, "But I have a map! Can you help me find it?"

The local responds, "Sure, let me take a look at your map."

The local studies the map for a moment and then says, "Ah, I see the problem. You've got your map upside down!"

The Talking Dog

A man walks into a bar with his dog and says to the bartender, "I'll have a beer and my dog will have a water."

The bartender looks at the dog and says, "Wow, that's a really well-trained dog! He can drink water!"

The man replies, "Well, that's not all he can do. Watch this." The man then turns to the dog and says, "What's on top of a house?"

The dog responds, "Roof."

The bartender is amazed and says, "That's incredible! Can he do any more tricks?"

The man nods and says, "Sure. Watch this." He then turns to the dog and says, "What's the opposite of black?"

The dog responds, "White."

The bartender is stunned and says, "That's amazing! How did you train him to do that?"

The man replies, "Well, I didn't exactly train him. He's actually a talking dog."

The bartender is skeptical and says, "A talking dog? That's ridiculous!"

The man then turns to the dog and says, "Okay, Rover, tell him about yourself."

The dog responds, "Well, I was born in a litter of talking dogs. My father was a talking dog, and my mother was a talking dog. I went to obedience school and then got a job as a translator for the United Nations. But I got bored with that, so I decided to go on the road with my owner and see the world."

The Forgetful Senior

An elderly man walks into a doctor's office and says, "Doc, you gotta help me. I keep forgetting things!"

The doctor nods sympathetically and asks, "How long have you been experiencing this?"

The man scratches his head and replies, "What?"

The Blonde and the Math Test

A blonde high school student walks into her math class and sees that there's a test that day. She didn't study and doesn't know anything about the subject. Panicked, she decides to cheat and sits next to the smartest guy in the class.

The test begins and the teacher hands out the papers. The blonde starts to copy her neighbor's answers when she notices that he keeps erasing and changing his answers. She leans over and whispers, "What's wrong? Why are you changing your answers?"

He responds, "I just realized that I got the first answer wrong, so I'm trying to fix it."

The blonde looks at him in disbelief and says, "Oh my gosh, you know the answers?!"

The Talking Dog

A man sees a sign outside a house that reads, "Talking Dog for Sale." Intrigued, he rings the doorbell and asks the owner if he can see the dog. The owner brings out a dog and says, "Go ahead, ask him anything."

Skeptical, the man asks the dog, "What's on top of a house?"

Without missing a beat, the dog responds, "Roof!"

The man, still not convinced, asks another question. "How does sandpaper feel?"

The dog replies, "Rough!"

Impressed, the man asks the owner how much he wants for the dog. The owner replies, "Ten dollars."

The man is taken aback and asks, "Why so cheap?"

The owner responds, "Because he's a liar! He never said any of those things!"

The Monkey's Paw

A man walks into a curio shop and notices a strange-looking monkey's paw on the counter. The shopkeeper explains that it has the power to grant three wishes to the person who holds it.

The man is skeptical but decides to give it a try. He holds the paw and wishes for a million dollars. Suddenly, he hears a loud knock on the door, and when he opens it, a delivery man hands him a check for one million dollars.

Thrilled, the man decides to make a second wish. He holds the paw and wishes for a beautiful mansion. Suddenly, he finds himself standing in front of a magnificent estate.

Feeling greedy, the man decides to make one final wish. He holds the paw and wishes for a beautiful wife. Suddenly, he hears a loud knock on the door and opens it to find his ex-wife standing there.

The Drunk Man and the Taxi Driver

A drunk man stumbles out of a bar and hails a taxi. He slurs his words and tells the driver to take him to the other side of town.

As they're driving, the man suddenly opens the door and starts to lean out. The taxi driver yells, "What are you doing?!"

The man responds, "Just giving the dog a break!"

Confused, the taxi driver looks around and sees no dog. He then realizes that the drunk man is talking about himself.

Exasperated, the driver pulls over and says, "Listen buddy, I can't take you any further if you keep doing that. You're going to get hurt."

The man apologizes and promises not to do it again. The driver starts driving again and they continue their journey.

A few minutes later, the man opens the door again

and starts to lean out. The driver yells, "What are you doing now?!"

The man responds, "Just checking to see if the dog made it across the street!"

Senior Citizen's Confusion

An elderly man walks into a doctor's office and tells the receptionist, "I need to see the doctor right away. It's an emergency!" The receptionist asks what's wrong, and the man replies, "I have a terrible case of diarrhea and I can't remember where the bathroom is!"

The Magic Mirror

A man walks into a bar and sees a sign that says, "We have a magic mirror. If you tell it a lie, you'll disappear."

Intrigued, the man walks up to the mirror and says, "I think I'm a millionaire." Poof! He disappears.

The bartender chuckles and says, "You're not a millionaire, are you?"

The man's voice from behind the mirror responds, "No, I guess not."

The Barber and the Lawyer

A barber and a lawyer are having a conversation. The lawyer says, "You know, I'm tired of people thinking that all lawyers are greedy and dishonest. We're not all like that."

The barber replies, "Yeah, I know what you mean. People think that all barbers are gossips and know everything about everyone."

Just then, a man walks into the barber shop and the barber whispers to the lawyer, "That's actually true, I do know everything about everyone."

The lawyer rolls his eyes and says, "And they say lawyers are the ones who can't keep a secret."

The Blind Man and the Cheese

A blind man walks into a grocery store and asks the clerk for some cheese. The clerk asks, "What kind of cheese would you like?"

The blind man responds, "I don't know. What do you have?"

The clerk says, "We have cheddar, Swiss, mozzarella, feta, blue cheese, and more."

The blind man thinks for a moment and says, "I'll take that one," pointing to a large wheel of cheese.

The clerk cuts a slice for the blind man and hands it to him. As the blind man takes a bite, he says, "Wow, that's the most delicious cheese I've ever tasted. What kind is it?"

The clerk replies, "It's a wheel of Swiss cheese."

The blind man smiles and says, "Great, I'll take the whole thing."

The clerk is surprised and asks, "Are you sure? It's a really big wheel of cheese."

The blind man responds, "Oh, I'm sure. I've been craving a good book to read."

The Genie and the Blondes

Three blondes were walking through the desert when they stumbled upon a magic lamp. They rubbed the lamp, and out popped a genie.

The genie said, "You each get one wish. What would you like?"

The first blonde said, "I want to be rich and live in a big mansion."

The genie snapped his fingers and said, "It is done."

The second blonde said, "I want to be even richer and live in an even bigger mansion."

The genie snapped his fingers and said, "It is done."

The third blonde thought for a moment and said, "I want my friends to be even richer and live in even bigger mansions."

The genie snapped his fingers and said, "It is done. But I have to ask, why didn't you wish for something for yourself?"

The third blonde replied, "Well, I've always wanted to be smart, but I figured if my friends were rich and successful, I'd learn from them."

The Horse Race

A man walked into a bar and saw a group of men sitting around a table. He asked them what they were doing, and they said they were having a horse race.

The man was intrigued and asked how the race worked. The men explained that they each had a horse and would simulate the race by jumping up and down and making horse noises.

The man thought this was ridiculous but decided to join in. They all jumped up and down and made horse noises, and the man's horse won the race.

The man was ecstatic and asked the others how much he had won. They said he had won $10,000.

The man was overjoyed and asked what he should do with his winnings. One of the men said, "Why don't you take your horse to a real race and see how it does?"

The man thought that was a great idea and went to the track. His horse came in last place.

The man went back to the bar and told the men what had happened. They all laughed and said, "You should have taken the saddle off!"

The Talking Dog

A man walks into a bar with his dog and orders a beer. The bartender is amazed when the dog says, "I'd like a beer too."

The bartender can't believe his ears and asks the man, "Is your dog really talking?"

The man replies, "Yes, he's a talking dog. I'll prove it to you."

The man turns to his dog and asks, "What's on top of a house?"

The dog replies, "Roof."

The bartender still can't believe it, so the man asks another question. "How does sandpaper feel?"

The dog responds, "Rough."

The bartender is thoroughly impressed and asks the man if he can buy the dog. The man replies, "No way! He's my best friend. But you can talk to him if you'd like."

The bartender leans down and asks the dog, "What's the best bar in town?"

The dog responds, "The one with the meat on the floor."

The Genie in the Bottle

An elderly man was walking along the beach when he found a bottle. He rubbed it and out popped a genie.

The genie said, "I will grant you three wishes, but be careful what you wish for."

The man thought for a moment and said, "For my first wish, I want to be rich."

The genie nodded and the man suddenly found himself surrounded by piles of money. Excitedly, he said, "For my second wish, I want to be young and healthy again."

The genie nodded again, and the man suddenly felt youthful and full of energy. With one wish left, he thought carefully and said, "For my final wish, I want to donate one of my kidneys to charity."

The Dyslexic Devil Worshipper

An elderly man goes to church every Sunday and one day he runs into his friend, who he hasn't seen in a long time.

The friend says, "Hey, I haven't seen you in church lately. What have you been up to?"

The man replies, "Well, I've been going to a different church."

The friend asks, "Oh really? Why did you switch?"

The man responds, "Well, I found out I'm a dyslexic devil worshipper. I was going to the Church of Santa, but I meant to go to the Church of Satan."

The Cursing Parrot

An elderly man goes to a pet store to buy a talking parrot. The owner of the pet store warns him that the parrot he's interested in has a bit of a foul mouth.

The man decides to buy the parrot anyway and takes it home. As soon as he gets home, the parrot starts swearing and cursing at him.

The man tries to get the parrot to stop, but it won't listen. Finally, in frustration, the man sticks the parrot in the freezer.

After a few minutes, the man starts to feel guilty and takes the parrot out of the freezer. The parrot is shivering and apologizes, "I'm so sorry for my behavior. I promise I won't curse again."

The man is amazed and asks, "What made you change your mind?"

The parrot responds, "When I was in the freezer, I saw a chicken with a really bad attitude."

The Stolen Car

A man walks out of a store and finds that his car has been stolen. He calls the police and reports the theft.

The police dispatcher asks, "Can you describe your car?"

The man replies, "It's a red convertible, with a white top, and it has a bumper sticker that says, 'I love Justin Bieber.'"

The police officer on the other end of the line pauses for a moment and then says, "Okay, we'll keep an eye out for the car. But I have to ask, are you sure you want it back?"

The Talking Parrot

A man buys a talking parrot from a pet store. The parrot seems to be quiet on the car ride home, but as soon as they enter the man's house, the parrot starts talking nonstop.

The man tries to ask the parrot questions, but the parrot just keeps talking. Finally, the man gets frustrated and yells at the parrot, "Shut up!"

The parrot stops talking and looks at the man. "Finally, you understand me," the parrot says.

The Mathematician and the Farmer

A mathematician and a farmer are having a conversation. The mathematician asks the farmer, "How many sheep do you have?"

The farmer replies, "I'm not sure. I never counted them."

The mathematician says, "Well, let's count them together."

They start counting, and after a while, the mathematician says, "There are 148 sheep."

The farmer is impressed and says, "Wow, you're exactly right. How did you do that?"

The mathematician smiles and says, "I used a simple algorithm. I counted the number of legs and divided by four."

The Three Elderly Ladies

Three elderly ladies were sitting on a park bench, enjoying the warm sun. Suddenly, a man in a trench coat ran up to them, opened his coat and flashed them.

The first lady had a stroke.

The second lady also had a stroke.

But the third lady's arm was too short to reach.

The Confused Parrot

A man bought a parrot and took it home. He spent hours trying to teach it to talk but it just wouldn't say anything.

One day, the man was sitting in his living room when the parrot suddenly spoke up, "What's for dinner?"

The man was overjoyed and immediately replied, "Chicken!"

The parrot just looked at him, puzzled. "Chicken?" it repeated. "What's that?"

The man was surprised but figured the parrot just needed a little more time to learn. So he took the parrot into the kitchen and showed it a raw chicken.

The parrot still looked confused. "What am I supposed to do with this?" it asked.

The man realized that he had accidentally bought a parrot that had been raised by vegetarians.

The Clever Lawyer

A man was on trial for stealing a loaf of bread. The prosecutor was trying to prove his guilt and asked a witness, "Did you see the man steal the bread?"

The witness replied, "No, but I saw him eating it."

The prosecutor thought he had the case in the bag, but the defense lawyer spoke up, "If my client was eating the bread, that means he must have bought it. How could he have stolen it if he paid for it?"

The prosecutor was stumped and the man was acquitted.

After the trial, the man asked his lawyer, "How did you come up with that argument? I didn't buy the bread."

The lawyer replied, "I know, but I didn't want to ask you to lie under oath."

The Mathematician's Bar Tab

A mathematician walks into a bar and orders ten beers.

The bartender looks at him and asks, "Ten beers? Are you having a party or something?"

The mathematician replies, "Oh no, I'm just really thirsty."

The bartender pours him ten beers and the mathematician proceeds to drink them all in rapid succession.

Impressed, the bartender asks, "Wow, you can really hold your liquor! How do you do it?"

The mathematician responds, "It's simple. I just use the principles of calculus to determine the exact volume of alcohol my body can handle and adjust my drinking accordingly."

The bartender nods in understanding and starts to calculate the mathematician's bar tab.

When he finally comes up with the total, he slides

the bill across the bar and says, "That'll be $100."

The mathematician looks at the bill and smiles. "Actually, according to my calculations, the limit of my bar tab as it approaches infinity is zero. So I don't owe you anything!"

The Amnesiac Chef

A chef wakes up in a hospital with amnesia. He can't remember who he is or what he does for a living.

The doctor comes in to check on him and asks, "Do you remember anything about yourself?"

The chef thinks for a moment and then says, "I remember cooking a delicious chicken dish, but I can't remember the recipe."

The doctor nods sympathetically and leaves the room.

A few minutes later, the doctor returns with a plate of chicken. "Is this the dish you were thinking of?" he asks.

The chef takes a bite and his eyes light up. "Yes, that's it!" he exclaims.

The doctor smiles and says, "Great, you're a chicken chef!"

The chef is thrilled to have his memory back and

starts making plans to open his own restaurant. But as he's leaving the hospital, he suddenly stops and turns to the doctor.

"Wait," he says, "what was that dish called again?"

The Magic Trampoline

A man walks into a store and asks the salesman, "Do you have a trampoline that can make me jump higher than my house?"

The salesman responds, "No sir, I'm sorry. We don't sell magic trampolines."

The man looks disappointed and asks, "Are you sure? My friend has one and he can jump over his house."

The salesman chuckles and says, "I'm sorry sir, but that's impossible. Trampolines can't make you jump higher than your house."

The man looks at the salesman and says, "Well, my friend must have a really small house then."

The Unlucky Golfer

A man goes golfing with his buddies one day, but he's having a terrible game. Every time he swings the club, he misses the ball completely.

After several holes of this, the man looks up at the sky and says, "God, please help me with my golf game. I'll do anything, just please help me."

Suddenly, a bolt of lightning comes down from the sky and strikes the man. His friends rush over to see if he's okay, and the man looks up at them and says, "Who's up there playing golf?"

The Perfect Husband

An elderly woman was asked, "What makes your husband the perfect man?"

The woman replied, "Well, he's never late for dinner. He's always attentive, he never argues, and he always cleans up after himself."

Impressed, the person asked, "Wow, how did you find such a perfect man?"

The woman replied, "Oh, I didn't find him. I trained him."

The Absent-Minded Professor

An absent-minded professor was on his way to an important meeting when he realized he had forgotten his laptop at home. He quickly turned around and rushed back home to retrieve it.

Once he arrived home, he realized he had left his laptop's charger at the office. So he quickly drove back to the office to grab it.

As he was driving back to the meeting, he realized he had left his phone at home. Frustrated and out of time, he pulled over to the side of the road and muttered to himself, "I can't go to a meeting without my phone, laptop, and charger. I'm not a complete idiot!"

Just then, he noticed his reflection in the car's side mirror and exclaimed, "Oh no, I left my car keys at home too!"

A Lawyer's Fate

A lawyer died and was standing in front of St. Peter at the gates of heaven. St. Peter looked at him and said, "You're not welcome here."

The lawyer was shocked and asked, "Why not? What have I done wrong?"

St. Peter replied, "Every time you entered a courtroom, people fell asleep. We can't risk that happening up here."

The lawyer was disappointed but didn't give up. "Please, St. Peter," he said. "Isn't there any way I can come in?"

St. Peter thought for a moment and said, "Well, we do have a different place for you. It's not quite heaven, but it's not quite hell either. It's called Purgatory."

The lawyer was hesitant but decided to take his chances. So he entered Purgatory and found himself in a beautiful garden with all the luxuries he could ever want.

He was happy for a while, but eventually, he grew bored and wanted to leave. So he went to St. Peter and said, "I've had enough of Purgatory. I want to go to hell."

St. Peter looked at him and said, "I'm sorry, but you've already passed that way."

The Broken Clock

An elderly couple were celebrating their 50th wedding anniversary when the husband decided to surprise his wife with a special gift. He went to the local clockmaker and commissioned a custom-made clock that played a melody every hour on the hour.

The clockmaker delivered the clock to the couple's home, and they were thrilled with it. However, the next day, the wife called the clockmaker and said, "The clock you made for us is broken. It plays a different tune every hour!"

The clockmaker was confused and asked the wife to describe what was happening. She said, "At one o'clock, it played 'Happy Birthday,' at two o'clock, it played 'Jingle Bells,' at three o'clock, it played 'Auld Lang Syne,' and so on!"

The clockmaker realized his mistake and apologized profusely. He explained that he must have mixed up the melodies while assembling the clock. He offered to fix it immediately and promised to deliver a new clock the next day.

The husband was understanding and said, "It's

okay, we can still enjoy the clock. It's like a surprise every hour!"

The wife disagreed and said, "No, I want it fixed! I don't want to be reminded of how many more birthdays I have to endure!"

The Dog's Advice

A man and his dog were walking in the park when the man suddenly asked the dog, "Do you think I'm a good person?"

The dog thought for a moment and said, "Well, you always feed me, take me for walks, and give me lots of love. I think you're a pretty good person."

The man smiled and said, "Thanks, buddy. That means a lot."

A few minutes later, the man asked the dog again, "Do you think I'm a smart person?"

The dog thought for a moment and said, "Well, you threw a stick for me to fetch, but then you ran after it yourself. I don't think that was very smart."

The man laughed and said, "You're right, buddy. Sometimes I do silly things."

As they continued their walk, the man asked the dog one more question. "Do you think I'm a handsome person?"

The dog looked up at him and said, "Well, let's put it this way. When we go for walks, other dogs don't seem to notice you."

The Forgetful Golfer

A golfer is playing a round with his friends when he suddenly stops and looks puzzled. "What's wrong?" asks one of his friends.

"I can't remember if I've played this hole before," says the golfer.

His friends reassure him and say, "Don't worry, you definitely played this hole last time we were here."

The golfer nods and takes his shot. As he's walking to the next hole, he suddenly stops again and looks confused.

"What's the matter?" asks his friend.

"I don't remember if I've played this hole before either," says the golfer.

His friends try to jog his memory and remind him of the last time they played, but the golfer is still unsure.

Finally, one of his friends suggests, "Why don't you just mark on your scorecard which holes you've played before?"

The golfer is relieved and thinks it's a great idea. He takes out his scorecard and starts marking an 'F' next to each hole he's played before.

As they approach the next hole, the golfer stops and looks puzzled again.

"What's wrong now?" asks his friend.

The golfer replies, "I can't remember if I got an F or a B on this one."

The Magic Trampoline

A man walks into a magic shop and asks the owner if he has any new products.

The owner says, "Yes, I have a brand new magic trampoline. It's guaranteed to make you jump higher than you ever have before."

The man is intrigued and decides to buy the trampoline. He takes it home and sets it up in his backyard.

Excited to try it out, he takes a running start and jumps onto the trampoline. Suddenly, he's soaring through the air higher than he's ever gone before. He's having the time of his life until he realizes he has no idea how to get down.

Panicking, he starts bouncing around trying to get back to the ground, but he just keeps going higher and higher. Eventually, he's so high up that he can see his entire neighborhood.

Just then, a man in a hot air balloon floats by and calls down to him, "Excuse me, do you know where I am?"

The man on the trampoline yells back, "Yes, you're in a hot air balloon!"

The man in the balloon responds, "You must be a magician!"

The man on the trampoline yells back, "No, but I do have a magic trampoline!"

The Generous Lawyer

A lawyer is at the Pearly Gates, waiting to be admitted to heaven. Saint Peter is looking through the book of life and frowns at the lawyer.

"I'm sorry," says Saint Peter, "but your name isn't in here. You're supposed to go to the other place."

The lawyer is shocked and asks, "But why? I've always tried to be a good person and help others."

Saint Peter thinks for a moment and says, "Well, I can't find any good deeds you've done, except for one. You once gave a dime to a homeless person."

The lawyer looks relieved and says, "Well, that's not much, but at least it's something."

Just then, an angel comes up to Saint Peter and whispers something in his ear.

Saint Peter's face turns red and he looks angry. "What's wrong?" asks the lawyer.

Saint Peter responds, "I just found out that that homeless person you gave a dime to was actually a billionaire in disguise!"

The Amish Elevator

An Amish family visited a big city for the first time and they were staying in a high-rise hotel. The father and son had never seen an elevator before and they were amazed by it.

As they watched people go in and out, an elderly woman stepped into the elevator. The Amish man turned to his son and said, "Quick, get the rope."

The woman overheard them and asked, "Excuse me, are you trying to hold the elevator for me?"

The Amish man replied, "No, we're going to pull it up for you."

The Genie and the Lawyer

A lawyer is walking along a beach when he finds a bottle. He opens it and out pops a genie. The genie says, "Thank you for freeing me. For your kindness, I will grant you one wish."

The lawyer thinks for a moment and says, "I wish for world peace."

The genie looks at him and says, "Are you serious? Do you know how difficult that would be? There are so many factors to consider - political, economic, social. It's just not possible. Do you have another wish?"

The lawyer thinks for a moment and says, "Okay, how about this? I wish that all the lawyers in the world were honest and ethical."

The genie thinks for a moment and then says, "So, you want world peace?"

The Broken Refrigerator

A man calls a repairman to fix his broken refrigerator. The repairman arrives and asks, "What seems to be the problem?"

The man replies, "It's not cooling properly. I think it might be the compressor."

The repairman opens the refrigerator door, takes a look, and says, "Hmm, I think I see the problem. Let me check something."

He then takes a can of beer out of the refrigerator, opens it, and sets it on the counter. After a few minutes, the beer starts to bubble and foam over.

The repairman says, "Yep, that's definitely the problem. You have a compressor issue."

The man is surprised and says, "Wait a minute, how did you know that from the beer?"

The repairman smiles and says, "It's simple. It's beer logic. If the beer is warm, the fridge isn't working."

The Hearing Aid

An elderly man goes to the doctor and complains about his hearing. The doctor gives him a hearing aid and tells him to come back in two weeks.

Two weeks later, the man returns to the doctor's office. The doctor asks, "How's your hearing now?"

The man replies, "I haven't picked up the hearing aid yet. I've been waiting for a quiet moment to go get it."

The Lumberjack

A lumberjack walks into a magical forest and starts chopping down trees. Suddenly, the forest nymph appears and says, "You can't chop down those trees! They're magical and will grant you three wishes if you spare them."

The lumberjack thinks about it and decides to spare the trees. The forest nymph disappears and the lumberjack goes back to his work.

A few hours later, the lumberjack gets thirsty and wishes for a cold drink. Suddenly, a bottle of cold water appears in his hand.

Impressed, the lumberjack decides to make his second wish. He wishes for a delicious sandwich, and just like before, it appears in his hand.

Excited, the lumberjack starts thinking about his third and final wish. He pauses for a moment and then looks around and says, "I wish for a road that leads to my house."

The forest nymph appears again and says, "Are you sure that's your final wish? You could wish for anything!"

The lumberjack replies, "Yes, I'm sure. I'm tired of hauling these trees all the way home."

Hearing aid malfunction

An elderly man walks into an audiologist's office with a concerned look on his face. He tells the audiologist, "My hearing aid isn't working properly. I can't hear anything out of my left ear."

The audiologist takes a look at the hearing aid and notices that it's clogged with earwax. She takes it apart, cleans it thoroughly, and puts it back together.

"Now, let's test it out," she says.

The audiologist claps her hands loudly and asks, "Can you hear that?"

The man nods his head and says, "Yes, I can hear you now."

The audiologist then claps her hands again, but this time covering her left ear. The man looks puzzled and says, "I can hear you just fine, why are you covering your ear?"

The audiologist replies, "Oh, I just wanted to see if your hearing aid was working better. It's a new feature that blocks out background noise."

The Magic Pill

An elderly man goes to see his doctor and complains about feeling tired all the time. The doctor asks him some questions and runs some tests, but can't find anything wrong with him.

Finally, the doctor says, "I have just the thing for you. It's a magic pill that will give you energy and make you feel young again. Take one every morning with water and you'll be good to go."

The man is skeptical but decides to give it a try. The next day, he takes the pill and feels great. He has energy he hasn't felt in years and is able to do all the things he used to do.

Excited by his newfound energy, he goes back to the doctor and says, "Doc, that pill was amazing. I feel like a new man. What's in it?"

The doctor smiles and says, "It's just a simple multivitamin. The magic is in believing."

www.ingramcontent.com/pod-product-compliance
Lightning Source LLC
Chambersburg PA
CBHW070659220526
45466CB00001B/504